CHRONIC BACK PAIN?
SAY GOODBYE

"The 60-Minute Solution"

Dr. David Light

About the Author

Since Dr. Light healed himself over two decades ago from a sports injury that left him debilitated with lower back pain, he's been fascinated by the Brain and the Mind.

He's been studying neuroscience and learning the ways and the powers we have to heal ourselves from many disorders.

In this book, he will share with you a step-by-step method to eliminate chronic lower back pain that he's been teaching for years to hundreds of his clients and patients. His goal is to share this with as many people as possible around the world.

There is a place for Medicine, but there's also a need to understand self-healing.

Contents

About the Author .... *i*

Introduction *1*

Chapter 1: 1986—My First Patient *2*

Chapter 2: The Brain—World's Largest Medicine Cabinet *6*

Chapter 3: Unlock the Pain—the Key Is O^2 .... *11*

Chapter 4: The Beginning of the End of Pain *17*

Chapter 5: Your "60-Minute Solution"—It Really Is Simple *21*

Chapter 6: Change the Messages—Change the Pictures *26*

Chapter 7: The Game—Your Road to Recovery *32*

Introduction

As you will read in the upcoming chapters, Dr. David Light practiced head and neck Orthopedics in N.Y. and trained many doctors in his proprietary method, a method he discovered over two decades ago. His therapies are exclusively geared toward allowing oxygen back to the muscles, the KEY to unlocking the pain.

This book is intended to serve as a resource and educational guide only. The author, or anyone involved in this book program, *will not* assume medical or legal responsibility for having this book's contents considered a prescription to anyone. Treatment of health disorders needs to be supervised by your physician or healthcare professional.

Chapter 1:
1986—My First Patient

Welcome to a program that can truly change your life. You're reading this book because your back hurts. In the following chapters, I will share a simple (and I do mean SIMPLE) 4-step solution that, if you follow, has shown the most successful results. My patients, and now you are looking for a pain-free life so *you* can go back to doing all the things that make you feel free and alive! With this program, all these results are possible.

You've been suffering back pain for weeks, months, maybe even years. Believe me, you're not alone. One out of three people experience lower back pain and pain that shoots up from the lower back, such as sciatica (SIGH-ATTICA). I was just like you, in constant pain from a back injury that was wrecking my life until I ventured outside conventional medicine and discovered a simple approach to healing that left me pain-free and whole again.

I call it the "60-Minute Solution." If you give me just one hour of your time, you can also be pain-free and back to normal. In this instructional book, I'll explain how your body works and tell you exactly **why your back still hurts.** This essential information can help you create your own "60-Minute Solution." Then, I'll teach you simple techniques that can end your suffering within a week and possibly even within the next hour. This book contains a lot of information, so it's okay if you need to take a break every now and then. We all have different attention spans, so if you need a breather along the way, please go ahead and take it. Find the pace that's right for you.

Now, before we get started, here's how my story started:

Believe it or not, my first patient was me. More than twenty-five years ago, while playing tennis, I jumped as high as I could to reach the ball. In mid-air, I twisted my entire pelvis. When I landed, every muscle in my lower back was swollen. A friend of mine had to help me up and rushed me to the nearest hospital. For nearly three weeks, I was in constant pain; even breathing was incredibly difficult for me. Every breath caused severe pain in my lower back muscles until the inflammation finally subsided. I was finally back to normal, or so I thought. I went back to my usual routine, thinking everything was fine. But weeks later, I suddenly developed stabbing pain in my lower back. First, these spasms would hit me once or twice a day. Then they started happening every hour, lasting so long that I was unable to see my patients or drive to and from work. That's when I started seeing a chiropractor.

When I showed no improvement after many visits, he suggested I take an MRI. From that moment on, my life began to fall apart. My chiropractor told me I had three herniated discs in my lower back and needed to see an orthopedic surgeon.

Driving back to Manhattan that day, I was in so much pain that I was forced to stop in the middle of traffic on the 59th Street Bridge and get out of my car. Desperate for relief, I grabbed onto the metal studs on the bridge to help me pull and stretch until I could drive on long enough to pull over into an emergency lane. I stretched out in the back seat until the pain finally subsided.

My next step was to consult the top two orthopedic surgeons in New York. These acclaimed doctors were the chief surgeons for professional sports teams. After individually examining me and reviewing my MRI, they told me my only option was back surgery, which is always risky. Even with a successful outcome, I would only be able to work part-time. I'd also have to give up tennis. I consulted another top orthopedist who confirmed their dire evaluation. But I wasn't willing to settle for a half-lived life or the risk of serious back surgery. I decided to take control of my back pain and my future. I read every book I could find on the subject, both traditional and less conventional in approach, and even personally met with some of the authors. I was amazed by the information and insight I gathered.

With the proper tools and techniques, each of us has the power to heal many of our back problems on our own. I became the living proof of that. Within four weeks, I was working full-time again and back on the tennis court, playing eight to ten hours a week. I knew I was on to something important, and I decided to devote myself to helping others suffering from chronic back pain.

Trained as a dentist, I sought out some of the world's top specialists in head and neck trauma and orthopedics for further study and training. Since then, for more than twenty years, I've seen thousands of patients and trained dozens of doctors in the successful treatment of back pain—without the use of drugs or surgery.

Sometimes, the hardest moments in life help us find our true purpose. That's what happened to me, and it led to my "60-Minute Solution." But before we get into that, there's something even more important we need to talk about—the brain. Healing doesn't start with the body; it begins with the brain. In the next chapter, you'll learn how your brain is like a medicine cabinet, holding everything you need to start feeling better. This is where the journey to recovery truly begins.

Chapter 2:
The Brain—World's Largest Medicine Cabinet

It's time to begin so you can make your own "60-Minute Solution." We're actually going to start with your brain instead of your back. The brain is quite a powerful organ—actually a muscle—and it holds the key to your speedy recovery. This complex muscle is also a memory bank with billions of inter-neuronal connections that allow us to perform millions of actions per second. What you may not realize, however, is that the brain is also the world's largest medicine cabinet. What do I mean by that?

In only fractions of a second, millions of chemicals that act like drugs or medicine are being released from our brains into our nervous system. Their purpose is to help our bodies function in an optimal way, but sometimes, our own thinking causes these chemicals to hurt instead of help us. I'll give you some examples of how this happens. You're probably familiar with the fight or flight reflex—our natural instinct to flee when faced with imminent danger. Suddenly, in the face of serious harm or death, we find that we can move faster than we ever thought possible. How does this happen? It happens with the release of one of the brain's miraculous drugs known as epinephrine (EPEE-NEF-RIN) or adrenaline. It takes only a single, instantaneous thought to trigger that release and pump adrenaline to our lower extremities, enabling us to run with unbelievable speed.

Physical activity or even a simple movement can trigger the release of different drugs from the brain. For example, exercise induces chemicals known as endorphins (EN-DOR-FINS) to flow from our brain throughout our body, affecting our mood in a positive way. That's how runners achieve what is known as the runner's high, the elation they generally feel when they regularly work out. In the same way, when runners interrupt their usual training routine for an extended period, they often experience runner's blues or mild depression. It happens because they are no longer signaling the brain to pump out mood-enhancing endorphins. Believe it or not, even facial expressions and other nonverbal gestures send signals to the brain to release a drug that can make us feel good or bad. The more we use that gesture or expression, the more we program our brain to secrete that particular drug. And remember, your brain is a memory bank, and how it's programmed depends entirely on you. We'll discuss more on this later.

Right now, I'd like to talk about the back pain that's brought us together. If you would, please back up in your mind to that life-changing moment when you first injured your back.

Maybe you bent over and felt a sudden sharp pain. Within seconds, or by the next day, you were flat on your back and couldn't move. Or it might have happened in a car accident, a fall down a flight of stairs, or playing sports. Perhaps it came on slowly and more gradually over a period of weeks or months. The thing is, how you hurt your back is not important. What matters is that you ended up in a doctor's office with intense pain. Your doctor probably prescribed you pills and suggested you have an X-ray or MRI taken. They probably told you to stay in bed for the next few days until the problem resolved itself. From that moment on, however, your life began to unravel from persistent pain.

Each one of you reading this book has gone through an experience similar to this. Now, here you are, months, maybe even years later, wondering why your pain is still there and why your life has never quite gotten back on track. Let me tell you why: From the moment you first injured your back and throughout your body's healing stages, which took weeks, you started believing that *There must be something wrong in there.* Without realizing it, you began sending the wrong signals to your brain, verbally and non-verbally. This is what I've discovered through my months of neuroscience research and study.

After a few weeks in continuous pain, you begin to unwittingly program your brain to consistently send the wrong chemicals to your muscles, which it's still doing to this day; hence, your pain. Now, the trick is to reprogram your brain to end your pain. This is the essence of the "60-Minute Solution."

By the time you reach the last chapter of this book, you'll have the tools and techniques to turn around your pain-encumbered life. Before we get to the heart of the program, I'm going to tell you one more story. A few years ago, on a flight back to New York from Fort Lauderdale, I was sitting next to a woman in her early thirties, accompanying her young son. She seemed to be in discomfort, and I noticed she was reading a book on back pain. It struck me that fate had placed us next to each other, and I mentioned my work in treating patients with back problems. *"If anyone can help me with this,"* she said, *"I would owe them my life."* She told me she'd been an aerobics instructor until she injured her back ten months earlier. She could no longer work, and her constant pain and complaining were causing her husband to grow distant. In short, her marriage was falling apart—all because of her back pain, for which she could find no cure.

The beauty of sitting on an airplane is that there are no cell phones or other distractions. For the next two hours, I had her undivided attention, and she had mine. Thus, I was able to explain how the brain's drugs—designed to help us—sometimes actually cripple us and how we must *"reprogram"* our brains to get rid of the pain for good. By the time we landed two hours later, she understood why she was still in so much pain and what she needed to do to get her life back to normal. Two weeks later, I received a note from this woman, thanking me for ending her pain and saving her marriage! She was teaching aerobics again. And her passion for life was back.

What I'd like us to do right now is take a flight of our own. Imagine you're sitting next to me, strapped in your seat. No cell phone, no distractions. And I mean no distractions because I want you to be rid of your pain as quickly as the woman on that flight from Fort Lauderdale. When our flight ends in less than an hour, you'll have your own "60-Minute Solution."

As we get ready to end our mental flight, I want you to keep that sense of peace and focus. But before we move on, let's talk about something that might still be troubling you—your pain. Just like the flight helped us shift from one place to another, there's a way to move past the pain that's been holding you down. It's not difficult, and it doesn't take long to understand. So, let's look at it closely, starting with your muscles, which often cause discomfort. Pain, especially in your back, is linked to how your muscles work—or sometimes don't work. The key to unlocking that pain is something simple: oxygen.

Chapter 3:
Unlock the Pain—the Key Is O^2

Let's talk about pain for a minute. Back pain comes from our muscles. Whether it's upper or lower back pain, the muscle is the source of our discomfort. Muscle tissue is made up of millions of fibers like lanes on a superhighway. These fibers contract and expand. It's true for all the muscles in our body. For example, the hamstring muscle along the back of the thigh has the same fiber makeup as the trapezius (TRAP-EASY-US) muscle in the shoulder. The sole function of these millions of fibers is to contract and stretch. That's how our muscles do their work. For example, when we want to pick up a book, we use the bicep muscle in our upper arm. When we lift a heavy book, we contract the muscle tighter than if we were picking up, say, a pencil. Even that pencil requires the muscle to contract, but not as much as the heavy book.

The difference is that the heavier the weight, the more muscle fibers we use within that muscle to carry the load. Again, the function of any muscle is to contract and expand — contract when we use it for a specific task and expand back to its normal length when we rest it. **Just like a rubber band, muscle fibers are elastic.**

I know this is pretty basic stuff, but please stay with me here because this is important. **We are coming to the true source of your back pain shortly.** The key to this muscle elasticity is a crucial molecule that circulates in the body called "O^2," which we all know and call 'Oxygen.'

Oxygen is the fuel for our muscles in the same way that gasoline is the fuel for our cars. If you turn the ignition key of your car and the gas tank is empty, the car won't start. The magic is that even if your tank has been empty for weeks or even months, the moment you put a little gas in your tank and turn the ignition key, your engine will come back to life. The same holds true for muscles. Our blood vessels are the pipes that carry oxygen to our muscles. The oxygen is carried via the red blood cells in the blood to the muscle fiber. **That oxygen allows the muscles to contract and expand,** not only when we are lifting objects but also when we are stretching, jumping, bending, sitting, getting up, and so on.

Now, please visualize this: On a microscopic level, the oxygen molecule, O^2, attaches itself to each fiber within the muscle. It allows the muscle to contract and expand in sync with all the other millions of fibers within that muscle. Without the oxygen reaching those muscles, it's like trying to start a car without gas in the tank. *In the case of muscle, the lack of oxygen turns the muscle from "elastic" to "plastic."* Please remember this. A muscle with sufficient oxygen is elastic , **while a muscle depleted of oxygen becomes "plastic," which means it cannot stretch.** This was my first discovery. Hang in there a bit longer, and you'll understand where I'm going with this. Like the blood vessels, the nervous system is also a complex super highway of nerve fibers that travel from our brain to our muscles. While the muscle is the source of our discomfort, these nerve fibers interpret the muscle pain, carrying messages back to the brain that allow us to experience or feel the pain.

This process is similar to how we experience other stimuli, such as heat, cold, and our sense of touch. The nerves transport messages back to the brain that allow us to feel the stimuli. In the case of a back injury, that stimulus is *pain*. Now, let us return to that first time you experienced pain in your back. Regardless of the circumstances or cause, it was traumatic to the muscles in your lower back and/or upper shoulder and neck region. As it happened, the trauma to the muscle sent messages through those millions of nerve fibers to the brain, which for you meant pain. When muscle trauma like this occurs, the brain reacts to initiate healing by supplying the traumatized area with a large amount of blood. Why? Remember that oxygen is carried to the muscles through red blood cells. The brain orders a large amount of blood to the trauma area to provide oxygen and other nutrients needed for healing. This sudden influx of blood causes swelling, which we call inflammation. Unfortunately, this swelling presses on the nerves surrounding the injured muscles, producing a knife-like, stabbing pain. This causes even more discomfort—pain that will last until the swelling goes down and the pressure on the nerves subsides.

This means that the inflammation is actually there to help you heal. Unfortunately, the pain we endure during those next few days or weeks of healing conditions us to believe that *there's something wrong in there.* This is the point when everything changes, both physically and, later on, emotionally. I want to repeat this very carefully so it sinks in. During those early days and weeks, as we live through that healing period, we start to believe that we have a handicap, that there is something wrong with us because we've been living with pain for so long. From this moment on, we stress every time we feel the pain. In a sense, we continually relive the pain, day and night, 24/7. This can go on for years, but you can stop it. Please digest the information we just discussed. If necessary, go back and read this paragraph again because you'll need a clear picture to fully understand the information that follows.

As life moves forward, every time we feel a sensation in that traumatized area, even just tightness, stiffness, or a sense of weakness, we reinforce the notion that something is definitely wrong with us. Our inner voice kicks in and says, *"It must be because nothing else hurts."* Reinforcing this for many hours, day after day, adds up to a lot of conditioning. We all know that continuously supporting and reinforcing our minds with good thoughts builds confidence and self-esteem. The same holds true with negative thoughts.

During your healing process, you were continually bombarding your brain with negative thoughts. At first, they were induced by real pain. Then, later, after the healing, these negative thoughts continue to be induced by conditioned reflexes or reactions you had to the original pain. If it had not been for this conditioning, that pain might have long ago disappeared. But it didn't, and that's what we have to change.

To repeat: *This conditioning started when you first received a negative verdict from your doctor.* Then people you know started telling you their bad back pain horror stories. You got all kinds of advice: *"Don't do this...don't do that."* All this constant negativity set off what I call the Conditioning Mechanism—or CM—in your brain. From that time on, even though you healed physiologically and the inflammation was gone, the CM programming was set in motion. This was my next discovery.

What we need to discuss now is muscles have memory, and through repetition, the CM continuously sends chemicals to "tighten" the muscle to protect it, which in turn causes oxygen depletion to the fibers within the muscle.

Understanding this mechanism is the key to achieving your "60-Minute Solution" and getting back to jogging, aerobics, gardening, playtime with your kids and grandkids, and all the other activities that are important to living a full and healthy life. Not only that but by the end of this book, you'll have a clearer understanding of how the mind-body connection works. You'll finally be in a position to heal yourself if and when another back incident occurs in your future, as I did after my tennis accident more than twenty years ago.

Now that you understand how the mind and body work together, it's time to move from understanding to action. Just knowing this won't ease your pain—you need to use the right techniques to start healing. In the next chapter, we'll focus on simple, practical steps you can take as part of your "60-Minute Solution." These methods will help retrain your brain and change how it feels pain. We'll start by looking at the pictures and memories stored in your mind and how they affect your body.

Chapter 4: The Beginning of the End of Pain

Now it's time to begin working one-on-one with you on your personal "60-Minute Solution." I'll show you the practical steps, techniques, and "sensory" exercises I discovered and tested on my patients that will put you back on track to living a pain-free life. Your personal solution begins with learning how to change the images in your brain—the pictures in your internal "digital camera." We all have one, with its own photo album of images impressed upon it over time. It takes millions of pictures every second. The more profound or intense the situation, the deeper and more vividly the image becomes locked in our memory bank.

The beauty of the human mind is that we can substitute old pictures for new ones. By helping you substitute your old pictures with new ones, I will enable you to accelerate your healing. First, I want you to close your eyes and visualize the digital camera in your mind. Can you see it? Good. Now, turn it on. Done? OK, open your eyes again. We're about to start changing some of the pictures you have in your mind.

As we discussed earlier, muscles are elastic, like rubber bands. When we decide to use a particular muscle, it contracts or gets shorter. When it's not being used, it's relaxed and naturally stretched out. So, work equals contraction—a tighter muscle. And rest equals a longer, relaxed muscle when it's back to normal. Now, using your internal digital camera, focus on this picture—your muscle at work, with thousands of micro-fibers meshing like millions of teeth sliding into each other in an intricate gearbox.

Do you have this picture in your mind? Excellent!

Now, visualize your muscle at rest in its expanded or elongated state. Good! Remember that a muscle is normally at rest ninety percent of the time. Resting is its usual state. Can you see your muscles relaxed and elongated? Terrific! Hold that image for a moment. Allow that visual to become embossed in your brain and your brain's memory. Now, visualize the bloodstream flowing to that muscle, delivering essential nutrients, most importantly oxygen, to replenish the muscle's depleted energy and, more importantly, allow it to do its function, contract, and expand, as we discussed earlier. Picture the molecules of oxygen as they work their way into the muscle. Keep in mind that this is only possible because the muscle is resting, expanded (opened), allowing the capillaries to feed the oxygen to the muscle. In this relaxed state, which you are photographing, the muscle is able to absorb the oxygen that's so essential to restore its function and energy. Got the picture? Fantastic!

If you didn't get that picture, here is another image for you to visualize. Picture a garden hose. You turn on the faucet, and the water flows freely from one end and comes out the other end. As you picture this, imagine someone suddenly stepping on that hose, stopping the flow of water. This is what happens when the muscle is at work and constricted, with the fibers pressed tightly together, blocking the flow of blood and oxygen. On the other hand, during the resting state, which is ninety percent of the time, no one is stepping on our hose or blocking the flow. There's a continuous inflow of oxygen, and the muscle has the opportunity to refuel and return to its elastic state.

Here's an exercise I'd like you to try. First, notice how comfortable your arm is right now in its resting position while you are not thinking about it or using it. Now, grab a pen or pencil or something just as light. Lift it with your elbow suspended in the air. It's just a pencil, right? But you'll notice that your arm starts to get tired within a minute or two. If it were something heavier, your arm would feel the tension within twenty to thirty seconds. That shows how quickly the oxygen gets depleted from our muscles while they are working. You can lower your arm and relax again.

Now, you understand the value of your muscle's resting position. Your muscles are replenishing oxygen, regaining its fuel, ninety percent of your twenty-four-hour day. It's important that you take a moment and imprint this information in your brain's memory bank so the techniques we discuss next work for you quickly.

Now that you understand how important it is for your muscles to rest and recover, let's think about a time when this didn't happen. Remember when you hurt your back? That injury caused your muscles to tense up, and they stayed that way. This constant tension made the pain last longer because your muscles couldn't get the break they needed. In the next chapter, we'll explore what exactly happened during that time and how it affected your body.

Chapter 5:
Your "60-Minute Solution"—
It Really Is Simple

Now, go to the gallery section of your brain's camera and scroll back to the picture when you injured your back. At that moment, the inflammation had started pressing on the injured muscles and the surrounding nerves. When these nerves were being compressed, their corresponding muscles contracted and remained contracted. This debilitating process—in which your muscles lived in a contracted state—went on in your back for days and weeks. While you clenched up, grimaced, and did all the other things we all do when we're hurting, you never gave your muscles a break! They couldn't get the normal rest time they were used to or needed.

As we discussed earlier, muscles have memory, and that continuous state of contraction caused your CM, or Conditioning Mechanism, to kick in and embed photos and visuals into your brain's memory bank. In other words, your back muscles went into a state that we all know and call *spasms*. Within weeks, you actually healed, and the inflammation was gone. But now, the pain you were living with was the simple spasms due to the muscle's conditioning memory. This is where the conditioning shifted from second to fifth gear. Your thought, *"There's something wrong with me because I'm hurting,"* was nothing more than those spasms. But the message you sent to your medicine cabinet (brain) was, *"Protect me. It hurts in there!"* By way of the nerves, your fears and worries about something wrong started a self-defeating conditioning between your brain and those muscles. To add to this vicious cycle, your doctors and physical therapists were telling you that something horrible was going on in there, forcing you to restrict your movements, reinforcing the bad news your brain was getting. Most damaging were the verbal and non-verbal messages you were communicating to your brain. In effect, your brain became confused by the conflicting signals, much like that game of telephone we played when we were kids. From then on, your brain continued to secrete chemicals intended to protect you and help you heal—chemicals that were no longer needed. These emergency drugs continued to flow, causing the muscle to continue to spasm. The spasms, in turn, slowed the flow of blood and oxygen to the muscle.

With its oxygen supply diminished, the depleted muscle created unending pain. **Why?** Because now the muscles in your lower back are in a "plastic" state. You can stretch a rubber band all day, but picture holding a 3-ply garbage bag. Now stretch it. What happens? You can stretch it slightly but a bit more, and it actually starts to tear. That is exactly what happens in your lower back muscle every time you use it to twist, to sit, to stand up or to lie down. Every time you make a move involving your lower back, you're causing **micro-tearing in the muscle fibers, *and that's very painful!***

This is happening all day long. Every time you make a move, you're tearing muscle fibers and re-inflaming the area.

This *muscle tearing* is the TRUE source of your pain, and once you understand and digest it, the solution to follow will be simple.

In other words, your worries and concerns were responsible for this vicious cycle, preventing you from being able to heal completely. I used to tell my patients, *"There really is no such thing as chronic pain, only chronic memory."* It's important to understand that we're talking only about our voluntary muscles, such as the biceps, hamstrings, and those in the upper and lower back. With these voluntary muscles, we can tell the brain what we need, whether it's to lift an object, run for our lives, or get an infusion of drugs from our medicine cabinet. With involuntary muscles, such as the heart muscle, you don't have to dictate to your brain—your brain does everything automatically.

If we had to tell our brain when, how often, and how much blood to pump to and from our heart every minute of the day, we'd be dead before we knew it. Fortunately, we don't have to do this.

But when it comes to our voluntary muscles like our lower back, biceps, and hamstrings, we dictate to our brain and tell it what we need, whether it's to lift something or the sudden need to run from danger. Unfortunately, this control we have can sometimes backfire if we think we have something wrong when we actually don't.

After everything we've discussed here, the crucial point for you to realize is that oxygen is the most important ingredient for your muscles to function elastically and painlessly. Still, because of this nasty CM, your oxygen is not getting there.

That's it for this phase of the program. Now, we're about to move into the final two phases. And now that you have this new understanding, you'll be amazed at how simple your solution is. Don't be confused by its simplicity. In the past, many of my patients would think, *"It's too easy...almost too easy to be true."* If a thought like that comes to your mind, just remember what Einstein said,

"The definition of genius is taking the complex
and making it simple."

Most things in life are truly simple once we have the correct information to process. Think about that first bike you got when you were a kid. At first glance, it looked extremely complex—the chains, the gears, the pedals, and all the bars that connect the wheels to the steering mechanism. Once your mom or dad showed you the basics, where to sit, how to steer, how to balance, and you put them into motion through repetition, you were racing around the block in no time. It's not much different with adults and automobiles.

A visit to an assembly line at an automobile factory reveals just how complex a vehicle is, with all its internal parts and mechanisms. All we need is a driving instructor to give us the proper instruction, and we learn to use and drive a car safely and efficiently like we were born to drive. It's the same with the human body and the brain. We were born to use it. The problem is no one gave us an owner's manual. That's what we're doing together here.

Of course, just as with the car, there are more pieces to this complex puzzle. But this is what you need to know to take off. At this point, I want to thank you for your patience in getting through so much information thus far and to let you know that you're almost home. The most important concept for you to grasp and the most important tools you need for your "60-Minute Solution" are just ahead. Are you ready? Let's go!

Chapter 6:
Change the Messages—
Change the Pictures

Here's the most crucial part of your "60-Minute Solution," the concept that's essential for you to grasp:

Everything, verbal and non-verbal, that you communicate to your brain has consequences—instant consequences. And the more you repeat those verbal and non-verbal reactions, the more ingrained and dramatic those consequences are. What do we mean by verbal reactions in the context of back pain? It is everything from *"ouch"* and *"Oh, my aching back"* to the moaning and groaning so many of us do when we're hurting. It doesn't even need to be actual words. Just the sounds are enough. Then I made my next discovery: **Our CM nonverbal response is even faster.**

What do I mean by the nonverbal response? These are **wincing, grimacing, rolling her eyes in pain and frustration,** and all the other gestures we make, consciously and unconsciously, in reaction to pain. Very profound! Up until this book, you've been doing many things that have been destructive for you in ways you've never realized. From this moment on, the tools I'm about to share with you will help you eliminate these ingrained habits, their destructive consequences, and your relentless pain.

Do you know that even in our sleep, we are continuously conditioning our minds? Believe it or not, the pain we suffer while awake can go on even in our sleep. In psychology, it's long been accepted that when we sleep, our dreams often express the thoughts and concerns that have troubled us most during our waking hours and now reside in our subconscious. For example, if we watch a horror movie, hear bad news, or have an argument before going to bed, chances are our dreams, however surreal, will reflect lingering fear, anxiety, or tension. In effect, our mind is up, and our brain is at work 24/7—even as we sleep. Unfortunately, when your deepest concern throughout the day has been your nagging back pain, your muscles are also up and working all night, even though they should be at rest. Our mind continues to respond according to the negative and unhealthy signals it's been receiving all day, to the detriment of our muscles.

This destructive cycle can be stopped, and you have the power to do it! First, you need to understand that during sleep, our muscles need to *be* at rest. When we go to bed, saying that we need to recharge our batteries, what we really mean is that we need to recharge our muscles. But that can only happen if the conditions are right. And through these final steps, you will learn how to control those conditions.

We are about to change every verbal expression—whether it's spoken out loud or by your not-so-silent inner voice, and every non-verbal gesture that you make, minute by minute, when you are in pain or, and this is my next discovery *when you are **about to** experience pain.* Remember, our brain, just like our muscles, has a powerful built-in memory bank. The good news is that only you have the power to determine what your memory will hold. Right now, all your pain-related memories and all their consequences are based on your past belief that something is wrong. You've trained your brain hundreds of times a day, for weeks and months, to remember that *"Something is wrong."* That's a tremendous amount of negative reinforcement.

To eliminate those negative thoughts and pictures, you are going to literally replace and change them in your mind's vault: the memory bank. To do this, you need to first replace the negative verbal and non-verbal with positive verbal and non-verbal. This will take real discipline and concentration on your part. Don't worry—we'll take it step by step. If you're genuinely committed to this, over the next couple of days to a week or so, you will see amazing results.

Two senses are important to discuss here. Our eyes are for everything we see, and our ears are for everything we hear.

Our sight interprets everything in our visual field, from objects right in front of us to 200 feet and further away. When we drive, we notice many different things simultaneously, which the brain interprets and allows us to make smart decisions, whether to change lanes or suddenly step on the brakes.

So, how do we use our sight when it comes to healing? I call this "THE GAME." You're about to play simple mind games (with your mind). Through repetition, you can influence your mind.

There is something specific you can do to accelerate and impact your healing process. If you put your hand in front of your eyes and create a symbol using your fingers that represents you are feeling great, that's all it takes. A thumbs-up is a familiar visual that describes everything is just fine. When you feel pain or stiffness, the thumbs-up negates and covers over with *"Everything is just fine."*

Remember, your brain works best with symbols and pictures, so here's what you do. Anytime you're doing your verbal and nonverbal exercise (managing internal and external thoughts and words), if you put two thumbs-up in front of your eyes, you're adding a new, additional component to the healing process because everything starts with the brain. When the brain "now sees" everything is fine, all the chemicals necessary for your healing are sent out through the nervous system. Remember, the chemicals are everything, and you are in control.

The more senses you use, the quicker you're erasing all the negative thoughts (the photos in your "internal camera") that you've been building up over the months, maybe years, and replacing them with positive ones, which equates to accelerated healing.

Doing these sensory exercises many times a day is easier compared to the alternative you have—going to your therapist. Imagine being stuck in traffic, going back and forth from the therapist's office, sitting ducks in the waiting room, and finally getting the treatment after hours spent on unnecessary waiting time. Compared to that, this multi-layered repetitive exercise is a simpler path.

Change for the mind—pivoting—is not easy, but play the game, and your results will be quick.

Putting a thumbs-up in front of your eyes 5, 10, 15, 100 times a day while saying out loud, *"Everything is great! My back is great! I feel great!"* will accelerate your healing, and that's why I've had patients and clients that literally, within hours were so much better. They weren't afraid to do it all. They were all in!

The other important sensory mechanism is your hearing. When you say things out loud, not only do the people next to you hear you, but you also hear your words, and these words travel instantly to the brain and get processed. So, everything you say has instant ramifications. By saying over and over again, *"I feel great, my back is great,"* you're speeding up your healing because your brain interprets that, and it does the rest.

Now that you understand how powerful words can be in supporting healing, it's time to take the next step. With this knowledge about the mind's impact on recovery, a practical approach will be introduced. In the following chapter, "The Game" will be shared—a simple and enjoyable way to help relax and make the most of the healing process over the next few days.

Chapter 7:
The Game—Your Road to Recovery

The four steps I mentioned at the beginning of the book are what I call "The Game." Its purpose is to help my patients relax, enjoy their next 2–5 days, and make the most of what I'm about to share with you right now.

Step 1: For the next two to five days, when you are alone, you are going to talk to yourself out loud several times a day. I know it sounds a bit strange. But what you're doing is having conversations with your mind. You'll tell your mind that everything is totally okay and that nothing is wrong with your back (or any other body part that hurts).

The most critical time to have these talks with your mind is when you actually experience the pain. But please do it during your normal periods as well, when the pain is absent. Right now, this minute, I want you to start playing the game. Talk aloud to your mind as if you are having a conversation with a good friend. Know that your mind hears everything you say. As you speak to it aloud, you'll also be changing what that little voice inside your head had to say to reinforce your past negative verbal remarks. That inner voice never stops talking and reinforcing, and you're going to change what it says. Right now, we're going to take a fifteen-second break while you have that brief conversation with your mind. As you're talking out loud, telling your mind that the pain does not mean a thing, that your back is fine, that *"I am OK,"* do your best to believe every word you say.

One final thought before we sum up this step. When actors are studying new lines for a film or TV series, they need to fit into their new characters. That requires their whole demeanor to change. They will follow the lines of the script and allow themselves to fall into their new character even if it contradicts their nature. They do it for one reason only—because they love it! You need to love it as well. The reward is days away, maybe sooner, maybe later. So, go ahead and start talking.

Take a 15-second break. Repeat "I am OK, I feel GREAT!" *Five times.*

Now that we're back, it wasn't so difficult, was it? Remember, *"It's just a game."* For these talks, I want you to find private moments as often as possible for the next two to five days as you replace negative thoughts and pictures in your head with good ones. I especially want you to have these conversations the moment you feel pain or think you're about to experience it. Ten to fifteen seconds of talking out loud daily will do. Ideally, you'll have these chats a hundred times a day. I know that sounds like a lot, but please remember that you have filled your picture album with thousands, if not millions, of pictures since your first painful episode. If you want to replace the whole album in a short period of time, you'll need to overcompensate. If you're committed to this, I know throughout your day, you can find a private place for many of these fifteen-second time-outs. We're not talking about hours a day here, but minutes. And I do believe you're worth it. Please keep visualizing the blood flowing to those muscles, oxygen penetrating deep into the muscle, and all the other past beliefs, and those visuals disappearing! This is most important.

In a short time, your pain will shrink in size and frequency, and you'll see how effective the game really is. For many years, I've had non-believers, and even the most skeptical, become my star players after finally letting go of their doubts and playing the game with true conviction. What gave them the drive to succeed at this? When their episodes of pain started to shrink in frequency, they began to smile, and their successes were genuinely profound. Everyone accomplishes their win at a different rate. But I've found that generally speaking, the harder your effort, the quicker the payoff. Remember, in the next few days, as you play the game in earnest, you'll be undoing the negative conditioning of months, maybe even years. The more you do it, the quicker you'll end your pain. The key is to make the commitment and stick to it.

Now, we're ready for **Step 2.** My second discovery was *"the power the corner of your lips and the corner of your eyes have on your mind."* This step is the non-verbal gesturing—all those facial gestures and other movements you make when you experience pain. A simple smile instead of a frown when you're feeling pain or discomfort in your lower back is all it takes to negate the chemicals that usually come, causing more pain. Instead, "healing chemicals" show up, allowing a flow of oxygen to the muscles in the back and releasing the muscle. Over a short time, through repetition, the pain will dissipate. Every time you smile or laugh when you start feeling pain, you're one step closer to being pain-free.

My third discovery is *"the moment before the pain."* After living with chronic pain for a while, your mind knows when the pain is coming, and the gestures on your face, specifically the corner of your lips and the corner of your eyes, go into frown mode just before the pain actually begins. From now on, every time you are about to bend down, climb stairs, or lift something, you're going to think of something positive, something that makes you happy inside and out, *and smile* BEFORE *the pain.* It might be Seinfeld's favorite moment. The memory of your first child being born. A beautiful sunset. A good joke. Anything that makes you laugh or anything that makes you smile. Let's try it.

Do something slowly that you're normally reluctant to do, such as getting up from your office chair. As you do it, think positive thoughts. Yes, even though you feel a little pain, it's okay. And, by the way, you might not feel pain this time, especially after you've been doing **Step 1** for a day or two. Don't be surprised. It simply means these sensory exercises are already starting to work!

You may experience that nothing is hurting when it usually does because of all the positive information you've been listening to. Remember, the brain is a sponge, and things happen fast when it's processing new information. If you still feel that nagging pain, remember, you're used to the pain anyway. Visualize that everything is okay in there, and the discomfort will diminish once you give it a chance. Nothing dramatic happens in an instant, but repetition will surprise you. All of a sudden, those muscles will free up in there. Their elastic nature will return, and you will feel so good!

Now, back to this exercise. Changing your gesture to a smile or even laughter will not make the pain worse. You'll be camouflaging the hurt with smiles and laughter. And that's the point. It's hard for the mind to register *"there is something wrong in there"* when you're smiling, especially when you're laughing hard. Yes, you really are in control of your mind, and please don't ever forget that.

Think about it for a moment: *How can Michael Jordan score sixty points in a game, even with a fever or a sprained ankle? How can an NFL player continue to play when he's injured?* They understand the power they have to camouflage the pain. Here's another example. If you took someone depressed and asked them to hold up a mirror to their face and force a smile, a huge smile, or, better yet, fake a laugh, you would see how fast their negative state would change, at least for the moment. I'm not saying that smiling and laughing as camouflage is a cure for depression. My point is you can't smile and be depressed at the same time in that one moment. The brain cannot send messages to your face and body to make you feel depressed, while your smile sends messages to it saying, *"No, I'm happy."* The same mechanism holds true for your pain. Now, we'll allow you a few seconds to do this. Okay, go ahead.

[Please take a 10-second break to let this all in]

Good! That's what you're going to do from now on each time you feel or anticipate pain as you reprogram your brain's memory pattern.

Now, it's time for **Step 3.** As you try the following exercise, you may find yourself laughing to yourself. That's okay—everybody does that when they first do it. Find a mirror and stand in front of it. I'd like you to make all the negative gestures in response to any pain that you can possibly think of. The brain is amazingly complex and clever. It reads all those gestures and interprets them accordingly: *"Oh my god! Something's wrong again!"* Yes, that's what you've been doing. Now that you understand where the vicious cycle of pain initiated from, you can understand the power you have by playing the game and by allowing the brain to do its thing once again and recharge your batteries. Every negative gesture you replace with a smile, a laugh, or a happy thought will tell the brain that nothing's wrong there. Even though you might have experienced pain, you've expressed to the brain that *"Everything is alright."* Just two to five consecutive days of this game, and you are on your way to recovery.

Let's take a practice run. As you face yourself in the mirror, make one of your patented gestures — the wince, the grimace, whatever it might be. Now, replace it with a positive response brought on by a happy thought. See how easy it is? Easy, simple, yet profoundly important for your recovery.

Time for **Step 4**! The more you do the steps above, the more you'll feel comfortable and confident about getting back on that tennis or basketball court that you've avoided for so long. Back when I had my injury, using the same steps that I'm sharing here with you, I decided to take the ultimate test after I began working full-time again, and my back pain had subsided. I returned to the tennis court for the first time in nearly a year. The moment I started hitting, the pain returned instantly, and it was worse than ever. I remember actually shaking, so I stopped playing. I tried to play again two or three times that week, but I realized that every time I stepped on the court, the intense pain was returning because I was reliving the most traumatic moment of my whole ten-month experience. We all know that a picture is worth a thousand words. But even more important, one episode in our mind is worth a thousand pictures. And I was reliving my most traumatic episode!

Those painful pictures I'd created in my mind that day, moments after jumping for that ball, were coming back bigger than ever. In essence, these pictures stored in my brain were the biggest and the brightest in vivid color. Of course, they were the most profound. This is what started my whole collapse. I decided it was my time to replace those pictures. I went back to the tennis court, but instead of playing, I just stood there. I closed my eyes and brought back pictures of myself playing and playing hard without pain. It wasn't that difficult since I'd played tennis many times for many years before that accident—without pain. I had those pictures tucked away somewhere in storage. It was just time to let them out and delete the bad ones. I remember standing on the court for three to four minutes with my eyes closed so as not to be distracted by the world around me. I focused on those great pictures I was playing in my head. Then I started hitting with my friend… in pain… through the pain. It hurt. Boy, did it hurt! Yet, I felt that if I kept going hard, the blood flow and the oxygen would do its thing. And that's what happened! Within minutes, the pain was leaving my system. To this day, I remember how great it felt. Overcoming that pain was the end for me—the end of the *pain*.

Now, you don't necessarily need to do this for yourself right away. But one day, you too will want to get back on the court or run on the beach or do whatever it is that you've been longing for. You can wait or go for it now. If you ever decide to do it, remember that those traumatic photos will come up for you bigger and brighter than the rest of those negative pictures you just tore up in your mind. It takes the focus and intensity I described a moment ago to make them disappear.

If getting back on the court is too big of a challenge for you, you can always reach out to me. I've been coaching athletes for years, and I'd be happy to help you get back to your active lifestyle.

Now that you know the four steps of this program, I want to give you a living example of the concept I just described. A number of motivational speakers give fire-walk seminars across the country. Imagine hundreds of men and women at these seminars walking barefoot on red-hot coals. And what's more, no one is rushed to the nearest hospital afterwards with third-degree burns on their feet. You'd think with something as searing hot as fiery coals, and everyone would be severely burned and in terrible pain. But they aren't. How is this possible?

What these trained speakers do to the audience prior to the fire walk is this. First, they program them for their big moment. For a two-hour period, they ingrain or brainwash them to understand that *"It's easy…the mind is powerful, and each and every one of you can do it."* Next, the speakers plant pictures in the mind of the audience—walking over the coals without feeling the heat. Three to four hours later, everyone is in line walking over the burning coals, and they don't feel it. I repeat: *Their feet do not feel the heat.* Believe me, I know—because I've done it myself. The speakers have embedded new pictures in their audience's minds temporarily. Just long enough so the coal-walkers could have the confidence and drive to come through it with flying colors and without pain or injury. To put it more simply, it's mind over matter.

Lastly, you may have been living with back pain for a few months or even years. Do you recall the example I gave at the start of this program comparing oxygen to gasoline for our car? I told you that it doesn't matter how long the gas tank was empty. With fresh gas in the tank, you can turn the key, and, like magic, the car fires up. The same holds true for you, as it did for me. Remember my story—how I desperately wanted to get back on the tennis court. You might not have a strong desire to work out daily or to play hours of tennis regularly. But your great accomplishment will be getting back to your normal life — lifting your child, working full-time, and driving long distances without pain.

I have one more favor to ask. Please go through this book more than once. Give it a good read a number of times. During your first run, there will be parts that hit close to home for you. You'll tend to focus on those and maybe miss out on other points. That's great because the ones you focus on will bring you to your next level of pain relief. But there are other parts in this book that you'll need to review so that you can go all the way with this program and get the most from it that you possibly can. Every component you focus on is a key to your ultimate healing, the process that will allow you to be rid of the pain for good. Remember, I was told I would need serious back surgery, but I decided to seek an alternative path to recovery. During my days of training, a very prominent doctor told me, and I quote, *"You pick your doctor, and you pick your therapy."* What did he mean by that?

Simply this. You can choose to go to a surgeon, or you can choose alternative treatments (self-healing). I chose my alternative. And now, years later, I'm on the tennis court eight to ten hours a week, playing the game I love and enjoying it as much as ever.

With this, our flight together ends, and we've just landed. Before we get off the plane, I'd like to return for a moment to the woman I encountered on that trip back from Fort Lauderdale, the aerobics instructor who had lived in pain for so long. Thanks to our two hours of uninterrupted time together, I was able to observe, critique, and finally eliminate every gesture—the squint of her eyes, every negative movement of her lips, and the shrug of her shoulders. She was able to rid herself of every painful episode she'd been experiencing until that very moment. During those two hours, I role-played, showing her how to prevent those gestures from ever returning. Changing what she said to herself every time she'd experienced the episode was her "60-Minute Solution." I can't tell you how rewarding it was for me to see her giggle and laugh every time I pointed out to her what she was doing to allow the pain to persist. She'd never realized that she'd been doing most of these things unconsciously for months. Most people don't.

Thank you so much for letting me have this time with you and for giving me the opportunity to be upfront and candid. I've given you the tools to achieve your recovery, and I'm confident that you'll get there. Finally, please realize that both conventional and non-conventional medicine has its place. It is up to you to be selective and decide when to choose one over the other.

In Conclusion: Consulting and coaching are powerful tools for health and healing. Just like top tennis and basketball players who work with coaches to improve their skills, anyone can benefit from expert guidance on their journey to wellness. This book has focused on helping you understand how to heal yourself, which is an important step in taking charge of your health.

Learning how your body works is key to unlocking your full potential. If you're looking for more knowledge or want to understand the healing process better, don't hesitate to reach out. My email address is below, and I'm here to help.

Just as entrepreneurs often hire coaches to help their businesses grow, anyone seeking better health can gain a lot from having an experienced guide. A coach can offer fresh ideas, motivate you, and help you overcome obstacles. Remember, asking for help shows strength. Embrace your journey toward better health—support is always available when you need it.